menopause

a self-care manual

by

Judy Costlow
María Cristina López
Mara Taub

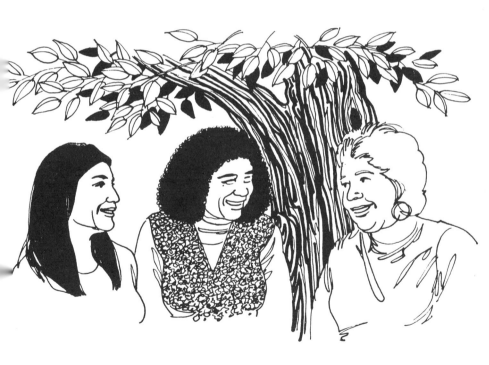

Illustrations by Lenndy McCullough

For permission to reproduce text or graphics from this book, write the Santa Fe Health Education Project, P.O.Box 577, Santa Fe, New Mexico 87504-0577. Telephone: (505) 982-3236.

The purpose of this book is to give support and resources, and to provide knowledge and information about women's bodies. It is not our intent to prescribe or to give medical advice.

The Santa Fe Health Education Project serves primarily Santa Fe and Northern New Mexico. We are an organization offering services in health education, advocacy, and organizing.

We were founded in 1975 to develop effective, self-help groups capable of solving local health problems. We believe that everyone should have access to good medical care. Good health is a right and not a privilege, and our services reflect this belief.

TABLE OF CONTENTS

ACKNOWLEDGEMENTS

Our thanks to the following people for support, advice, and information: our editor, Patricia A. D'Andrea, who had hot flashes the whole time she was creating a complete first draft of this book; Cathryn Reed Poukey, who did the typesetting and assisted in design of the 1989 edition; the authors of the original edition: Edith Adams, Judy Costlow, Jeanne Gladfelter, María Cristina López, Maggie Morrison, and Pita Romero; illustrator of original edition and page 6 of this edition, Betsy James; the readers of this edition: Helayne Abrams, Kitty Barragato, Blythe Brennan, Theresa Clarkson, Kathleen Costlow, Kristin Eppler, Matt Kelly, Tracey Kimball, Julia Rosa López-Emslie, Mary Mokler, Marmika, Pauline Nuñez-Morales, Mary Parker, Lydia Pendley, Caryl Rodriguez, Gloria Ruiz, Sylvia Sedillo, Judith Swarth, Maria Luisa Taub, and Nadine Taub; board members not already mentioned: Ida Friedland, Jessica Doyle, Marta Gallegos, Orphelita Griego, Carmen Martinez Lieurance, Carla López, Corrina Lucero, and Lucia Trujillo; Ken Luboff, of John Muir Publications, and Marian Davidson for advice and encouragement; Amadea Morningstar, who read and added to the self-help sections; librarian at St. Vincent's Hospital, Jane Knowles; and everyone who helped with the first edition of this book.

INTRODUCTION TO THE REVISED EDITION

In l980 we felt that it was important to make more information available to women concerning the menopausal years. Now, in l989, we feel it is important to add to what we originally wrote.

The Santa Fe Health Education Project has been studying, learning, and teaching about menopause for over 10 years. We have continued to give menopause workshops throughout this time, and continue to learn from the women who participate in them. It is more than ever our feeling that women themselves are the greatest resources for learning about menopause. From workshop participants we have learned about their concerns at the menopausal time of life. Osteoporosis is one concern; breast cancer is another. Therefore, we feel it is important to include information on these topics. Our experience has also led us to believe it is important to expand our sections on nutrition and our material on hormone replacement therapy.

We believe strongly that menopause is a natural part of women's lives. Therefore, we no longer believe it is correct to call the physical sensations and changes that women may experience during those years "symptoms." We were inconsistent on this point in our original edition. In this one, we deliberately use the words "sign" or "complaint" or "discomfort," rather than continuing the implication that menopause is in any way a disease that has "symptoms."

For the past year, we have begun our menopause workshops by asking each participant to tell us who the person is that she most admires. The answer–overwhelmingly, and totally unexpectedly– has been "my mother." We believe this carries an important message. At the same time that many of us have worries and concerns over what menopause will be like for us, we are very much aware of the strength, productivity, and wisdom of older women—we admire them and want to be like them. The good news is, given time, we can be!

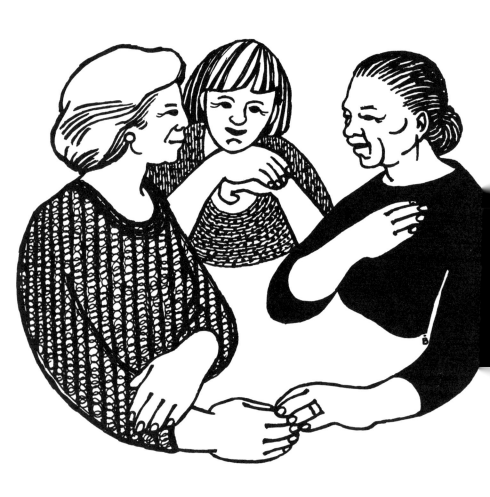

INTRODUCTION TO THE ORIGINAL EDITION

Menopause, a natural phase of a woman's life, has too long been ignored, talked about in whispers, or mentioned with pity and sympathy. It is time for all of us to speak out about menopause. This period of our lives can be frustrating, embarrassing, uncomfortable, and downright unpleasant. It can also be a time to become excited about our future, to be free of the demands and the worry of children, to be relieved of the bother of menstruation. It can be a time of discovery, of realizing our capabilities, and sometimes of embarking on a new career.

The Santa Fe Health Education Project, a private, non-profit, tax-exempt organization, became involved in menopause research and workshops through our monthly, bilingual (Spanish-English) health newsletters. In April 1977, we published a newsletter on "Menopause and Estrogen." The response from women in our state was tremendous. Many women called us seeking more information because, in general, the material available on menopause was inadequate. We were overwhelmed by the intensity of their questions and by their need to talk to other women.

Since information was not available, we thought that the best place to obtain it was from the women themselves. We knew that we could all learn together through research, exploring our own feelings, and discussing the social expectations of middle-aged women in our society.

A training group of six women was organized. The group included both Hispanics and Anglos who had either finished menopause, were going through it, or were about to start. There was a five-week training program that covered all aspects of menopause, with women doing the research and presenting their findings to the other members of the group. They developed skills in group presentations, research techniques, leading discussions of personal experiences, and learning how to conduct workshops for other women. After training, these women went into various New Mexico communities to conduct one-day workshops. This booklet is the result of those workshops.

To broaden our understanding of what women experience during menopause, we prepared a questionnaire. The questionnaires were first distributed at the International Women's Conference (May 1977) in Albuquerque, New Mexico and then to the women in our menopause workshops. We found the results of the questionnaires to be very informative because of the varied ages and backgrounds of the respondents. Answers came from women all over the state with an age span of 40 years between the oldest and youngest. Briefly, we are going to discuss some of the responses received from the questionnaires and workshops, and we want to show how the responses reinforced our thoughts that more information and discussion about menopause are needed. Perhaps, some of the responses will give you ideas for your workshop.

The questionnaire shows that most of the women who responded had some knowledge about the physiological changes during menopause. When asked, "What is menopause to you?" the main responses were: 1) It is a natural life-cycle; 2) It is the end of childbearing; and 3) It is the end of menstruation. Quite a few referred to the hormonal changes taking place in the body. Their knowledge about the physiology of menopause was very different from their feelings about it. While most of the women understood that menopause is a natural life-cycle that all women go through at a certain time, many of them still had negative feelings about it. A full 30 percent of those responding to our questionnaire said they dreaded menopause or associated it with a crisis, and these feelings seemed to be based largely on the kinds of information they had received.

Many women first heard about menopause as young girls from their mothers. Often women had seen their mothers going through menopause and this was their exposure. Other common sources of information were schools and doctors. Some women heard about menopause when they learned about menstruation. Although some of the women said that the information they received was detailed and informative, a majority of the women said that what they had learned was sketchy, and about 25 percent said they had heard very negative things about it. The questionnaire therefore indicates that most of the women who dread menopause do so because of the severe symptoms about which they have heard. However, only 10 percent of the women going through menopause have symptoms severe enough to interrupt their daily routine. Some symptoms may cause discomfort for a while, but are not severe. Many of the symptoms are similar to those some women experience during menstruation. Other women have no symptoms at all. Many women, especially those now going through or having gone through menopause, view this age as a liberating time of life. As one woman put it, "Menopause is the end of the reproductive but not the productive. A new freedom!"

We know that sometimes menopause can be a frustrating time for a woman. She may find herself snapping at her family, feeling that she is getting old or displaying some other emotional or physical change. When she speaks to her doctor (often a man who never will go through menopause), she may not find a sympathetic ear. Some women have suggested sitting down with their husbands and children to discuss menopause. This can be beneficial both to the woman and her family. Others have found the menopause workshops we have held to be a great place to air out feelings, questions, and anxieties.

The workshop discussions are a good time for women to talk about everything having to do with menopause. Dialogue among women who have gone through menopause and those who have not clarify many questions and alleviate many fears. We hope that with the help of this booklet and the workshops, people will understand that menopause is a natural experience. It can at times cause discomfort, and in some cases severe problems, but it can also be a gratifying and freeing experience. When we asked in our questionnaires if the women thought there was need for more information about menopause, 80 percent answered yes. We hope this booklet will be a first step towards answering the questions, stating the facts, and stimulating thought about this time of life.

Remember, menopause is not the beginning of aging, for from birth onward we are getting older. Some women think of menopause as a blossoming. Margaret Mead, the famous anthropologist, said she had more energy and felt better physically than ever before. She called it PMZ, Post-Menopausal-Zest.

Female Reproductive Organs

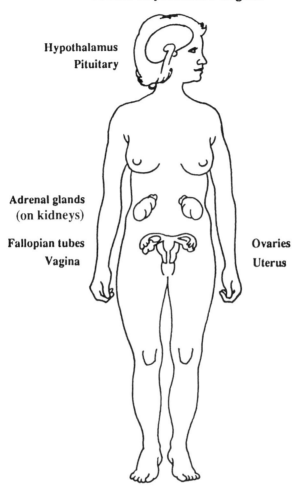

Hypothalamus
Pituitary

Adrenal glands
(on kidneys)

Fallopian tubes
Vagina

Ovaries
Uterus

Estrogen Levels During a Woman's Life

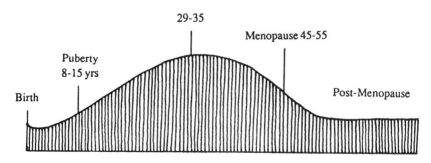

29-35

Menopause 45-55

Puberty
8-15 yrs

Birth

Post-Menopause

Chapter 1

ANATOMY AND PHYSIOLOGY OF MENOPAUSE

What is Menopause?

Menopause is that period in a woman's life when menstruation becomes sporadic and eventually ceases, fewer sex hormones (estrogen and progesterone) are produced, and fertility ends. It is a natural part of the aging process.

Every woman is born with a number of hormones in her body. These hormones are chemicals that carry messages from one part of the body to another and therefore influence all body functions. For example, the hormone insulin is sent from the pancreas to all the cells in the body to help them use sugar.

One of the important hormones a female child is born with is estrogen. As the child gets older the level of estrogen in her body increases until, at puberty, signals are passed from the hypothalamus to the pituitary gland (both located at the base of the brain) and they in turn signal the ovaries to start the menstrual cycle. A woman's hormone levels increase until she is between her late 20's and her mid-30's and then her estrogen levels begin a slow decline. This decline signals the start of some of the menopausal signs that many women experience.

When a woman is near age 50, her estrogen may reach a level which is too low to maintain her regular menstrual cycle. This is menopause.

Estrogen levels remain low for the rest of a woman's life, once she has entered menopause, but she is never without estrogen. Before menopause, estrogen is manufactured in the ovaries; after menopause, it is manufactured in the adrenal gland., the fat cells, and a small amount from the ovaries.

During menopause, a woman's ovaries stop producing a monthly egg, and decrease the cyclic supply of estrogen. A woman's periods change; they may be scantier, shorter, or further apart, or they may also be heavier, longer, or closer together. Sometimes a woman's periods may not come for several months. Because a woman may still produce an egg occasionally, she should use a birth control method for at least 2 years after menstruation stops if she does not wish to become pregnant.

Menopause usually occurs between the ages of 48 and 52. Participants who have attended our menopause workshops reported, however, that they had stopped their periods as early as 35 years old and as late as 60 years old. The best guideline for a woman to use to anticipate when she might go through menopause is to find out when her mother went through it. If her mother started menopause at an early age, it is likely that she will too.

It is not necessarily true that the younger a woman is when she starts to menstruate, the younger she will be when her menopause begins. It is also not true that the older she was when she started to menstruate, the older she will be when she begins menopause. Finally, there is no correlation between painful periods and childbirth and a woman's experience during menopause.

There is a laboratory test for menopause. The test does not measure estrogen production, it measures the levels of two reproductive hormones—Follicle Stimulating Hormone (FSH) and Luteinizing Hormone (LH). While estrogen levels decrease gradually over a period of years, FSH and LH levels increase markedly until after menopause.

Induced Menopause

"Induced menopause" is menopause that is brought on by outside influences. For example, induced menopause can occur as a result of various medical treatments, such as radiation and chemotherapy.

The most common cause of induced menopause is surgery. Surgical menopause occurs when a woman's ovaries, which produce estrogen, are removed before she has gone through menopause. In surgical menopause, a woman's periods stop and she may have menopausal signs. Because of the sudden change in hormonal balance, there might be discomfort until her body adjusts to the new situation. Women are often pressured to take estrogen; however, we suggest that a woman wait to see how she feels after the surgery before making a decision to take hormones, especially since women's reactions to surgical menopause vary.

If only one ovary is removed, and a woman has her uterus intact, she can continue to have periods. If her uterus is removed, she will not have periods any longer, whether or not her ovaries are removed. There is evidence that if even a small amount of ovarian tissue remains, sufficient estrogen may still be produced so there is no sudden change in hormonal level. The woman might experience menopausal signs, such as hot flashes, later in life.

Many physicians apparently do not believe that women over 40 need their ovaries. This is the reason why so many women who have hysterectomies also have their ovaries removed. We agree with the following legitimate reasons for removing the ovaries:

"The legitimate reasons for removal of the ovaries include: ovarian cancer, which is a relatively rare disease; certain hormone-dependent cancers of the breast and other organs; and highly cystic or otherwise benignly diseased ovaries. In the last instance, however, there is rarely need to remove both ovaries."
(Seaman; see References)

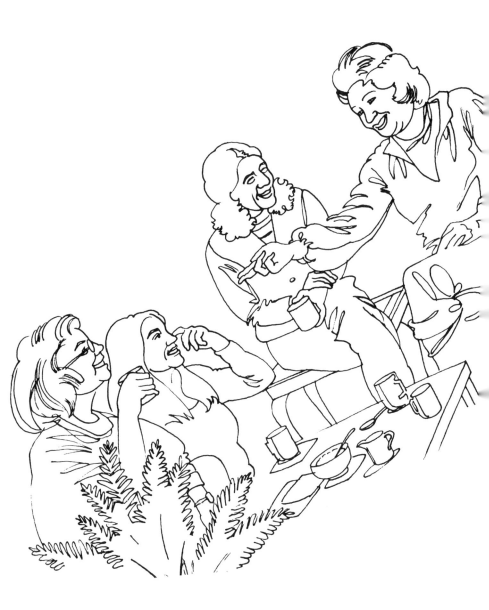

Chapter 2
SIGNS AND COMPLAINTS
OF MENOPAUSE

Personal Experience

It was a freezing December night in 1975 when I lay in bed, dreading to get up and go down a long cold hall to an even colder bathroom. Then, I had a hot flash and all of a sudden it was very easy to leave my warm bed! For the rest of the winter, I used my night-time hot flashes in this way. It made my friends laugh when I told the story of how I found out that hot flashes are not necessarily all bad! And now in 1989, I still have hot flashes— milder and fewer--almost every night.

The signs of menopause can appear at any time, especially between the ages of 35 to 50, the 15 years of hormonal transition. Some of the most common signs women experience during meno- pause are: hot flashes, chills, night sweats, palpitations, dizziness, headaches, pain, numbness in legs, weight gain, pimples, fatigue, insomnia, depression, anxiety, nervousness, oversensitivity, forget- fulness, irritability, tearfulness, and lethargy. Other complaints sometimes mentioned are itching on the bottoms of the feet, hearing problems, and indigestion, to name just a few. In addition, some women may notice a change in vaginal moisture.

There is no way to predict who will or will not have menopause signs. During menopause, approximately 80% of women will have one or more signs or complaints, 10% will have severe complaints that interrupt their daily routine, and 10% will have none at all.

Hot flashes are the sign most commonly associated with meno- pause. They are flushes of heat which sweep over the upper part of the body; they can last from a few seconds to several minutes. A red face, red blotches on the face and neck, sweating, and a feeling of suffoca- tion are four signs associated with hot flashes. They can all occur separately or together, and may happen as many as 30 times a day.

They may take place for a few weeks or continue for years. In most cases, these signs stop within a year or two.

What causes hot flashes? The cause is not understood, but this much is known: a hot flash is due to vasomotor instability, which is a rapid change in the diameter of the blood vessels. Estrogen is known to raise body temperature and progesterone to lower it. During menopause there are irregular levels of these hormones in the blood stream.

Dryness is a change that may occur in a woman's vagina as she gets older. A decrease in moisture and a loss of elasticity in some cases can make intercourse painful. There may also be vaginal itching and burning.

Women may encounter other problems after menopause, such as arteriosclerosis and osteoporosis. Arteriosclerosis, or hardening of the arteries, contributes to heart disease. Women usually have no problem with this disease before menopause, but after menopause women seem to get arteriosclerosis as often as men. Osteoporosis is discussed in Chapter 7.

Worries at Menopause

Menopause is a milestone in a woman's life, a reminder that she is past the halfway mark. It is also a time when relatives and friends may begin to die. No wonder menopause is sometimes hard to accept—coming to grips with death is not an easy process.

Menopause is a time of body change and also, often, a time of intensified feelings. Among those feelings may be a sense of loss as children leave home and intimate relationships change. A woman may have feelings of isolation, overwhelming exhaustion, inability to find purpose, and depression characterized by mood swings, a general loss of interest in life, forgetfulness and general mental distress. Many women have similar feelings and experiences; the woman who has such feelings is not alone nor is she crazy.

One of the most common worries women talk about in relation to menopause is the fear of "losing my mind." There is a myth that women have more mental breakdowns during menopause. "My aunt went crazy because of menopause." The fact is that the suicide rate of women in their teens and 20's is much higher than the suicide rate of women at menopause. Women in their forties and fifties generally report feeling more in control of their lives than ever before. Because menopause is a period of change, it is highly stressful. Women with good general health will get through times of stress with fewer adverse effects. Women who have learned to take care of themselves as well as they take care of others will probably have a less stressful time in menopause than others will.

One of the most helpful things a woman can do for herself to deal with any uncomfortable signs of menopause is to accept the experience rather than reject or deny it. Menopause comes to all women— those living alone, those who live with others, women who are lesbians, women who are heterosexual, women who are celibate, who are sexually active, who have children, who do not have children. Menopause comes to poor women, rich women, rural women, urban women, to those who are prepared and to those who are surprised.

Sex
Many women wonder if their experience with sex will be different during and after menopause. At the workshops the Santa Fe Health Education Project has given, some women report that they have always enjoyed sex and, because they no longer have to think about getting pregnant, it's even better for them after menopause. Because women's sexual responses do not diminish with age, a woman who had multiple orgasms when she was younger can continue to have them during and after menopause. Other women told us that they lost interest in sex after menopause. Maybe, they said, it is because sex is for having children and they can't have children anymore. Some women said that they never enjoyed sex in the first place and menopause did not make any difference. In other words, there is no "normal" pattern for sexual reactions during or after menopause.

Sex during menopause can be stressful because a woman's periods may be irregular, pregnancy may be less desirable, the birth control pill is less safe to use, and she does not know exactly when

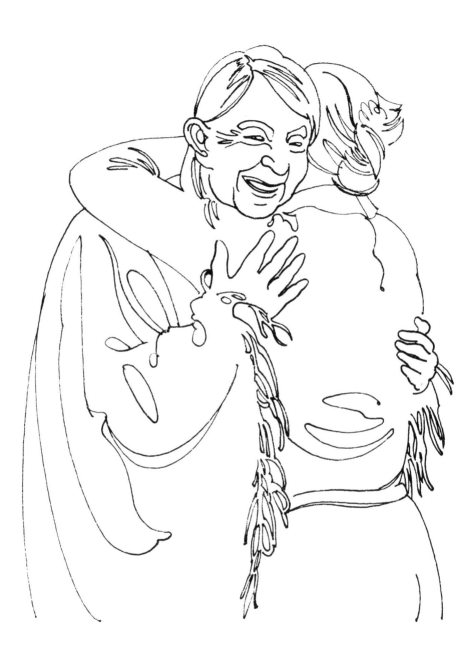

fertility stops. Of course, menopause is different for women who have had hysterectomies, since there is no possibility of their getting pregnant.

Treatment of Women

There are a number of body changes that occur as women age, particularly during the menopausal years; many of them are public and affect the way women are treated. Body changes include: skin changes, hair changes, breast changes, vaginal changes, weight changes, and eye changes. As at puberty, such changes are not immediately pleasant, and no matter what you do, they happen anyway. For example, too few people regard getting gray hair as positive.

Since women's life experiences teach them over and over that appearance is extremely important, times of change in appearance can create personal crises. The world treats women in their 50's differently, and for the most part even less respectfully, than women in their 20's, because of their differences in appearance.

In today's world, generally speaking, women have relatively little control over their lives. Tremendous inequities in the treatment of women continue to exist. For example, the United Nations recently reported that women do two-thirds of the world's work and receive only one-tenth of the pay. One has only to look at the corporate boardrooms, legislatures, and media conference rooms to know that women of 50, 60, 70, 80, and beyond are not represented in those places of power. Women often don't even earn a living wage.

In the past 20 years, the experiences of women have shown that there are possibilities for improving their lives. By talking and working together, women can have more life choices, believe in themselves, and become more powerful.

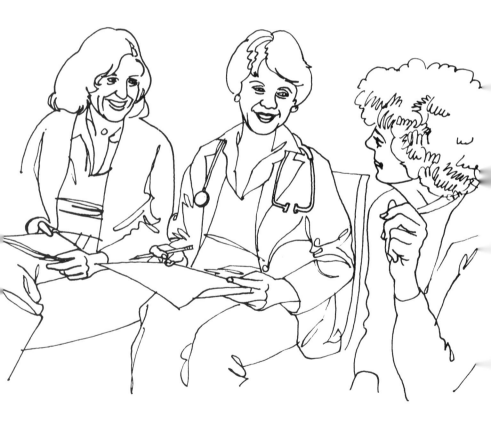

Chapter 3

MAKING HEALTH CARE DECISIONS

We believe health care decisions are each woman's responsibility, not that of some "expert." It is dangerous to believe everything "experts" say without question, because "experts" can never know a person as well as she knows herself, or care as much. It was experts who advocated the use of diethystilbestrol (DES) for pregnant women, the Dalkon shield as a contraceptive, and frequent dental x-rays for everyone. All of these procedures are now considered dangerous. DES caused cancer in both mothers and offspring; the Dalkon shield caused sterility and death; and dental x-rays caused salivary gland cancer.

Of course, experts can be useful as part of the decision-making process. But every woman has to put together different kinds of information—her knowledge of her body as a whole, her life history, and her judgment of possible treatments and their effects—in order to make wise health care decisions for herself. There are many helpful healing philosophies and techniques. Women need to be willing to learn healing methods which may not be familiar to them. A helpful source of information might be people who have followed a treatment that is being considered.

In evaluating a treatment, a woman needs to ask: What is its success rate? How is this rate known? Is the treatment permanent (such as surgery)? Is it systemic (affecting the whole body), as in chemotherapy and hormonal therapy? Is it cumulative (staying in the body and increasing with each treatment), as in radiation? Can its effects be harmful, and how? Are there less drastic treatments available? What will happen if the recommended treatment is not followed? How is this known?

In evaluating studies recommending a treatment, a woman needs to ask who paid for the studies and who will benefit from their conclusions. One example of a suspect study is a lung cancer study done by cigarette manufacturers. Other questions a woman needs to ask are: How many people were involved as subjects in the study? Over how long a period of time did the study take place? (Because many serious effects take a number of years to develop, 20 years is a reasonable amount of time to evaluate a treatment.) And finally, were so-called "side-effects" considered? How?

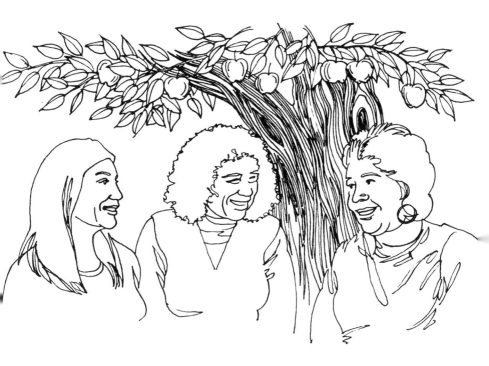

Chapter 4
HORMONE REPLACEMENT THERAPY

Personal Story

I dreaded menopause because I had always heard bad stories about it and also because it would mean the end of child-bearing, and I had never been able to have a child. At the age of 45, when my periods became irregular and I started having chills and hot flashes, I happened to read an article on Estrogen Replacement Therapy. I asked my gynecologist about it and she prescribed Premarin on a cycle of 3 weeks on and one week off. Within a week, the chills and hot flashes stopped. I continued to take Premarin for the next 8 years. I tried to stop four different times, but my symptoms were so severe that I went back to it. Later, I read about the danger of uterine cancer from ERT and, on my 60th birthday, decided to stop once and for all. The chills and hot flashes returned, but now, after 6 months, they are slowly lessening.

(10 years later she told us the continuation of her story)

Five years ago at age 65 I noticed spotting and knew something was wrong and realized it was something serious. After about six months, I saw a doctor and was found to have endometrial cancer. I had my ovaries, tubes and uterus removed. I had to go through radiation all that summer, out of which came uncontrollable diarrhea every morning which has continued for the 5 years since.

Many women take estrogen and other hormones—they are under tremendous pressure to do so. Women have been the subjects of experiments using hormones for many years, yet time and time again, women have found that what was hailed as a cure-all in one generation is found to be dangerous in the next generation. This is true of hormone therapies.

The use of hormones in the treatment of menopause has a long and controversial history. Estrogen and progesterone (two of the female sex hormones) were first isolated in 1923. Experiments performed in 1932, in which rats were given estrogen, showed that the rats developed breast cancer. Nevertheless, in the 1930's estrogen treatment in

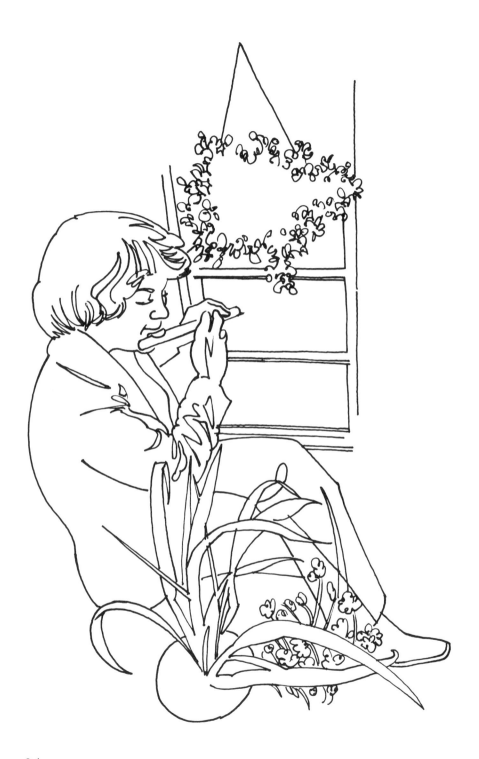

the form of diethystilbestrol (DES) was marketed. It was used to prevent miscarriages. Although later it was found that DES did not prevent miscarriages, it did cause cancer in some of the children born to women who had used DES during their pregnancies. DES was also used to dry up breast milk in new mothers, and to treat menopausal signs. The use of this treatment for menopausal signs increased slowly but steadily over the next 30 years.

In 1965, a book called *Feminine Forever* by Robert Wilson, M.D., promoted the use of estrogen to "keep women looking young forever." Even at this time there had been some research showing a possible link between estrogen use and endometrial cancer (cancer of the lining of the uterus), but these warnings were ignored. Women, pushed by their doctors, began using Estrogen Replacement Therapy (ERT) in record numbers. They were using a form of estrogen that is made from pregnant mares' urine under the brand name of Premarin.

In 1975, studies were published showing that estrogen users were 6 to 14 times more likely to develop endometrial cancer than non-users. The use of estrogen dropped dramatically. At the same time, drug companies which manufactured estrogen increased their efforts to find an alternative medication for menopausal women.

The drug companies' answer was to add progesterone to the estrogen. This treatment mimics the natural menstrual cycle and causes withdrawal bleeding. This "new" combination is now called Hormone Replacement Therapy (HRT) and is promoted as being "safe," and essential for the prevention of osteoporosis.

The taking of estrogen has been shown to decrease bone loss in women after menopause. However, estrogen users are at high risk for endometrial cancer and gall bladder disease. Some researchers have suggested that the use of progesterone decreases the hazards of estrogen alone. But "there is no acceptable evidence that adding progestogens decreases the risk of endometrial cancer." *(National Institutes of Health Consensus Development Conference on Osteoporosis, 1984; see References)* If women take progesterone with estrogen, they may be at risk for heart disease and strokes as well as other, yet unknown, dangerous effects. "There is concern that as more time goes by since the mid-sixties, when menopausal estrogen use became

popular, there may be more studies showing a link to breast cancer."
(Health Letter, Vol. 3, No. 6, see References)

Because there have not yet been long term (20 years or more) studies done with large numbers of women, Hormone Replacement Therapy (HRT)—estrogen and progesterone together—must still be considered experimental, at best. If HRT is thought of in this way, it will be easier to judge the risks versus the benefits of using HRT, despite the often misleading, high-pressure tactics which are frequently used to encourage women to take hormones. Remember, women over 40 are a large market in a consumer-oriented society. Somebody makes a lot of money when women buy so-called antidotes to the normal aging process.

Prescriptions for both Estrogen Replacement Therapy (ERT) and Hormone Replacement Therapy (HRT) have risen dramatically since 1981. Estrogen Replacement Therapy is still used sometimes because the progesterone in HRT may produce effects such as swollen, tender breasts, abdominal bloating, headaches, and depression in some women. HRT also causes monthly bleeding. In addition, many women go back on estrogen when their menopausal signs return after they had stopped taking it. Finally, because endometrial cancer can be successfully treated if caught in time, many doctors decide that the benefits of taking estrogen outweigh the risks.

Estrogen is prescribed in birth control pills as well as in Hormone Replacement Therapy. The cumulative effect of taking estrogen, no matter what the form or the dose, is not known.

If a woman is considering ERT or HRT, or if she is already taking it, she should be aware of these guidelines:
1. There are at least three groups of women for whom ERT is not recommended: women who have a family history of cancer, women with recurrent cysts and women with a history of blood clots. ERT is also usually not prescribed for patients with kidney or liver disease, enlargement of the lining of the uterus, and endometriosis or fibroids. The doctor should take a careful history and do a thorough physical examination including a Pap smear before prescribing ERT or HRT.

2. A woman needs to understand the risks of the treatment, as well as the benefits. If the doctor does not seem cautious with these potentially dangerous drugs, she should seek the opinion of another doctor.

3. A woman needs to weigh carefully what ERT can do *for* her as opposed to what it can do *to* her. Can she learn to live with her signs? If she remembers that the signs will go away eventually, perhaps she can be more tolerant.

4. During ERT, periodic examinations are necessary to check on the effects of the drug, to decide whether the dosage should be changed, and to evaluate the need for continuing therapy. *The aim is to take the smallest dose for the shortest period of time.*

5. A woman needs to discuss with her doctor the merits of a trial period without estrogen. She should also consider the possibility of a lower dosage.

6. The cyclic method of taking estrogen seems to be the best. This means that the woman takes estrogen pills for a 20- to 25-day cycle, then stops taking them for 5 to 7 days. This will help avoid possible harmful effects of prolonged, uninterrupted ERT. If more than a year goes by and the doctor has not suggested a trial period without medication, the woman should suggest it.

7. Taking ERT in pill form is better than taking it in weekly or monthly injections. The effects of ERT last longer when it is given by injection or through a skin patch. Women who are having vaginal discomfort during intercourse because of dryness and thinning tissue can use estrogen creams and suppositories. This form of estrogen, although not taken orally, can still be absorbed into the system of the woman or her partner, and its long-term effects on the body are not known. Therefore, as with all estrogen products, the cream or suppository should be used cautiously.

Some women use cocoa butter, coconut oil, sesame oil, and water soluable lubricating jelly such as K-Y Jelly as lubricants during intercourse to alleviate pain and irritation. Sometimes vaginal dryness can be reduced in other ways. The vagina is a muscle, and like any other muscle, it needs to be exercised to keep its tone. Included in Chapter 9, Self-Help, is a series of exercises that women can begin early in life to maintain vaginal muscle tone and to prolong their enjoyment of intercourse.

Personal story

I gave birth to my third and last child at age 40 and went back to work right away. My periods resumed their normal flow, but I soon began having severe hot flashes. I also had trouble sleeping at night and described my worst symptom as "feeling as though I had an irritant in my blood stream that made me feel prickly all over." My gynecologist did not at first think I was going through menopause, but he gave me an estrogen level or fertility lab test (I'm not sure which kind) and was convinced. He started me on Premarin in a cycle of 3 weeks on and one week off medication. After about 6 weeks, I noticed that all my symptoms had eased up. I continued to take Premarin for about 4 years. My physician was very cautious and conservative and always decreased dosage whenever signs lessened. By the age of 45, all symptoms as well as monthly periods, had ceased. I am now 62, and I have never had a recurrence of any of my symptoms.

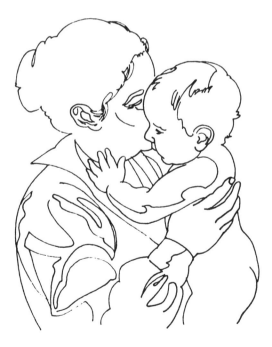

Chapter 5
CONTRACEPTION, STERILIZATION, HYSTERECTOMY

Personal Story

I was 40, and my children were 16, 13, 11, and nearly 9 when my youngest child was born. I had not planned on having more children and when I found out I was pregnant again, after all this time, I was quite dismayed. At first, all I could think about was 'starting over' with diapers, night feedings and being tied down again. I had gone to work as a substitute teacher after my youngest child entered second grade and I was enjoying my new-found freedom and the luxury of earning extra money. Having another baby now meant an end to this new way of life and a return to daily child-care. After a few weeks of feeling sorry for myself and looking at the 'work and bother' aspect of having a new baby, a strange thing happened. I began to look at the positive things a new life brings into a home—a new beginning, being needed, a new life to love and care for, another chance to try to do better at parenting, the first smile, the first tooth, sitting, crawling, the first step. I began to feel excited and happy at the prospect of a new little one to love. From that time on the pregnancy was a happy time of planning and waiting. I decided to give up my outside activities and really concentrate on enjoying this 'last' child. When my child, a girl, was born, the whole family pitched in to help and the homecoming was a happy occasion. The older children had cleaned the house and set the table for a party. The baby was a happy, healthy child who fit right into the family as if she had always been there, and the other children loved helping out with her. My 'late' baby turned out to be a blessing for me and my entire family.

It is possible for a woman to become pregnant during menopause. Although her periods may be scanty and irregular, an egg is still released occasionally. The medical approach to middle-aged pregnancy is essentially negative, stressing the risks of complicated pregnancies and birth defects. However, many pregnancies of middle-aged women are happy experiences. Early prenatal care, good nutrition and exercise are the best insurance for a safe and happy pregnancy and birth at any age.

CONTRACEPTION

For women who do not want to get pregnant, continued use of birth control for at least 2 years after menstruation stops is recommended. Birth control for women in their 40's and 50's is a subject which has been neglected; most of the emphasis today is on contraceptive methods for teenagers, and women in their 20's and 30's.

Methods

Contraceptive methods can only meet manufacturers' claims if used correctly, and may fail. Follow the directions. Ask questions.

The Diaphragm is effective if it is fitted correctly, inserted correctly, and always used with a spermicidal cream or jelly. Many women are choosing this method of contraception because of the absence of harmful effects.

The Contraceptive Sponge is said to be as effective as the diaphragm *only* for women who have never had any children. It comes in one size and can be bought over the counter without a prescription.

The Cervical Cap can be as effective as the diaphragm if properly fitted, but it only comes in four sizes, so a woman has to be sure that she is one of those sizes. Caps have been used in Europe for over 30 years, but in this country they are not approved for marketing as contraceptives. They can be acquired at some women's clinics, public health clinics or college health clinics.

Fertility awareness methods such as **rhythm** or the **Billings method** are thought to be less effective during the menopausal years because the changes taking place in the menstrual cycle make it more difficult for a woman to know when she is ovulating.

The Condom, a male contraceptive used with vaginal spermicidal foam, is very effective, and lessens the risk of sexually transmitted diseases.

Abortion is a method used to end a pregnancy.

Not Recommended

The Pill increases the risk of heart attacks in women over 40. Women on the pill cannot tell whether menopause has begun because they continue to menstruate.

The Intrauterine Device (IUD) may cause bleeding or spotting. Since these are also symptoms of uterine cancer, it is important not to mask them in any way. Because there are many other problems with IUD's, most IUD's are no longer available. They are now considered too dangerous for women of any age.

STERILIZATION, OR PERMANENT BIRTH CONTROL

Tubal sterilization involves blocking the oviducts, also called the fallopian tubes, in some way to prevent sperm and ovum from uniting. The following are examples of tubal sterilization:

Abdominal Tubal Ligation or "tying the tubes" is an operation which involves general anesthesia, a horizontal incision about 5 inches long in the lower abdomen, and 3 to 5 days of recovery in the hospital. During this operation, a piece of each oviduct is cut out and the ends are tied.

Laparoscopic Sterilization is another method of sealing the oviducts, and it is a faster and cheaper surgical procedure than tubal ligation. It is performed in a hospital, usually under general anesthesia, takes about 30 minutes and, if all goes well, the woman can leave the hospital in a few hours. Because such small incisions (two) are made, it is sometimes called the "Bandaid" method.

In 2.5 out of 1,000 tubal ligations and laparoscopic sterilizations, the tubes remain open, and the woman may become pregnant. Also, a woman should not undergo this operation thinking that it is reversible (that the tubes can be put back together), for it has been almost impossible, up to now, to rejoin the tubes. A sterilization is a difficult procedure. It is therefore essential for a woman to choose a doctor who has had considerable experience with this operation.

Many women who have undergone tubal sterilizations have reported some effects, like severe cramping and heavier periods, that were not mentioned before the operation. Some women said they would not have had the sterilization if they had known about these other effects. Studies are now being done to document the problems women have been reporting.

Vasectomy is a sterilization procedure for men. This operation is usually performed in a doctor's office under local anesthesia, and takes about 15 minutes. An incision is made on each side of the scrotum. The *vas deferens* (the tubes through which the sperm travels) are then cut and the ends tied. The man can leave the doctor's office after a short rest. This procedure should not be undertaken with the idea that it is reversible.

HYSTERECTOMY

A section on hysterectomy is included in this book about menopause because during a menopause workshop women asked why hysterectomies had not been discussed. They said, "I thought every woman had to have one as part of menopause." No wonder they thought this—50% of all women age 65 or older in the U.S. have had a hysterectomy.

The word hysterectomy is often used, but not always understood. *(See Chapter 1, on Induced Menopause)* It is important to know what is being done to you to be able to understand how your body will function in the future. Physicians call removal of the ovaries oophorectomy and removal of the fallopian tubes, salpingectomy.

There are many things a woman should consider and question before she agrees to a hysterectomy. She needs to understand that a hysterectomy is major abdominal surgery and carries such risks as problems with anesthesia, shock, or hemorrhage. Also, its long-range effects on health and longevity are not known. Each year, approximately 800 women die from hysterectomies, and some of these operations were unnecessary.

Along with the physical risks involved in this surgery, some women experience strong psychological reactions, for example, some sorrow and depression at the loss of female body parts.

As with any major surgery, especially surgery in which a part of the body is removed, a woman should get a second opinion before she makes a decision. It is also important to talk it over with family and friends. If the woman feels that it may be helpful, she has the right to take a friend with her to the medical consultation.

Reasons to Have a Hysterectomy

1. Cancer of the cervix or of the lining of the uterus.
2. Many large fibroids (benign tumors) on the uterus.
3. Heavy bleeding that does not respond to hormone treatments or to a D&C (Dilation and Curettage—the scraping out of the lining of the uterus), or when these treatments cannot be used for a particular woman.
4. When the tubes or ovaries are diseased and the uterus must also be removed.
5. Cancer of the uterus.
6. Complications in childbirth requiring removal of the uterus to save the mother's life.

Today in the United States, there are close to half a million hysterectomies performed each year. This is three times the rate of hysterectomies performed in England. This operation is very uncommon in Europe, where medical care is generally not based on a fee-for-service system. Unfortunately, some gynecologists perform hysterectomies for the purpose of sterilization or to forestall what they may consider to be future problems. The rationale behind this practice is that if a woman has "enough" children, she doesn't "need" a uterus and if the uterus is taken out, she won't have to worry about getting uterine cancer. A woman who is considering sterilization should find out about the alternatives available. Tubal ligation, for example, is less dangerous than a hysterectomy. *A hysterectomy should never be used for simple sterilization.*

When a woman has a hysterectomy after age 40, often her ovaries are automatically removed without her consent or any discussion. A woman should always discuss this issue with her doctor before surgery, keeping in mind that ovaries should never be removed without compelling and specific reasons. (Chapter 1, on Induced Menopause)

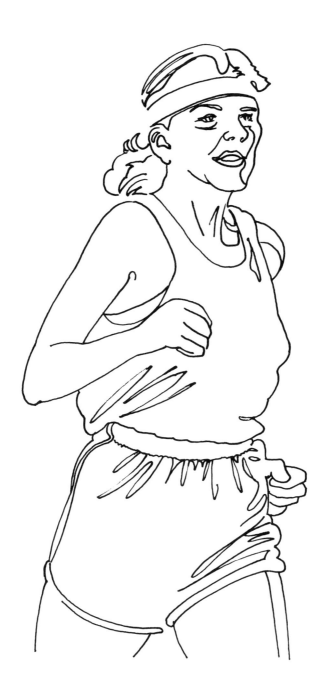

Chapter 6
OSTEOPOROSIS

A new "disease" has been added to the list of problems women in their 40's through 80's must confront. Osteoporosis, meaning porous or brittle bones, has been turned into a fashionable disease. This condition is due to the loss of bone mass as people get older and can become a problem if it is the cause of fractures. Generally speaking, older women and men have more broken bones than younger people, older women have more fractures than older men, and whites have more fractures than blacks.

People's bodies change as they get older. For example, skin may wrinkle and hair may turn gray. Everyone starts losing bone mass after age 35, and bone loss in women increases slightly after menopause. Twenty-five percent of all white women in the United States will suffer from fractures due to osteoporosis.

Effects of Osteoporosis

Although it is normal for a person's bones to thin as she or he ages, many people notice little or no change as a result of thinning bones. However, some people experience "crush" fractures of the vertebrae—the small bones that make up the spinal column in the back. This is one of the main causes of older people losing height. These "crush" fractures can also cause back pain, especially pain in the lower back. Another common example of crush fractures is the hump some older people get on the upper back.

Osteoporosis can also lead to broken bones in the arms, legs, wrists, and the hips. On occasion, bones may break during routine activities such as bending, lifting, or rising from a chair or bed. Fractures can lead to other serious problems such as pneumonia and bone infections.

Creation of a "New" Disease

Women over 40 are a growing percentage of the population, and at the same time, it is not socially desirable to be an "older" woman.

Creating a disease out of the normal process of bone thinning presupposes a "cure." Thus osteoporosis is making money for drug manufacturing companies which through advertising campaigns push calcium and hormones, and high technology businesses which push x-rays. Women over 40 are an increasingly large market segment, and are vulnerable to pressure.

Minimizing the Effects of Osteoporosis

Consuming sufficient calcium at times of heavy bodily demands for calcium such as the years our bones are growing the most—our teenage years, during pregnancy, and while nursing—is most important. "Although bone density continues to increase until people are in their mid-30's, the years of childhood and adolescence are the now-or-never years for building a strong skeleton." *(Health Letter, June 1987, see References)* However, eating healthy foods and exercising at any age can help strengthen bones.

How a person eats—especially if she tries crash diets, or junk or processed foods with lots of chemicals in them over a long period of time—can increase the effect of osteoporosis. Eating a variety of foods can minimize its effects. This means especially eating a lot of different whole grains (complex carbohydrates), low fat dairy products, and fresh vegetables, especially dark green leafy vegetables.

Boron, a trace element, has been found to have a positive effect on the rate of bone formation from calcium. Increasing boron in the diet of some women resulted in a decline of lost calcium and magnesium (in the urine) and an increase in blood levels of estrogen and progesterone. Boron is found in apples, pears, grapes, nuts, legumes and many vegetables. *(Study conducted by the Human Nutrition Research Center of the U.S. Department of Agriculture)*

Weight-bearing exercises—which involve both muscular contraction and the pull of gravity—can increase bone thickness if done regularly and frequently. Examples of weight-bearing exercises are: walking, jogging, bicycling, hiking, running, square dancing, cross-country skiing, and jumping rope. To be effective, these must be done for a minimum of 20 minutes, at least three times a week. Half an hour four times a week is more effective. Inactivity results in bone loss.

Smoking interferes with the way bones absorb calcium. To minimize the effects of osteoporosis, it is better not to smoke. Excessive alcohol consumption also affects how the body uses calcium. That is why it seems reasonable to drink only moderate amounts of alcohol, no more than one drink a day.

The British Medical Journal calls osteoporosis a "disease of affluence" as it is found mainly in countries, like the United States, where work no longer requires much physical exercise for many people, and where a lot of animal protein and processed foods are eaten.

Controversial Treatments for Osteoporosis

Hormone Replacement Therapy (HRT) is a controversial "treatment" for osteoporosis. *(See Chapter 4.)*

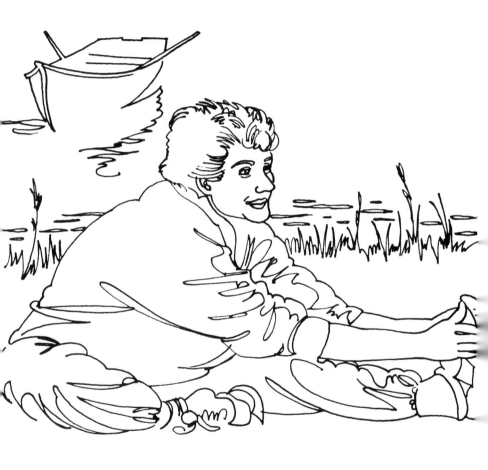

Chapter 7
BREAST CANCER

Breast cancer is included in this menopause book because many women associate breast cancer with getting older. In fact, breast cancer does affect many women over 40. Breast cancer is both common and frightening. One out of every 10 women is diagnosed with breast cancer at some time in her life.

What is breast cancer?

All body cells have a purpose; for example, skin cells make skin act like skin, and stomach cells make stomachs function properly. Cancerous cells, however, have lost their ability to do their job. They reproduce rapidly and spread to other parts of the body. *Dorland's Illustrated Medical Dictionary* (1981) says cancer is "a cellular tumor the natural course of which is fatal."

There are many different kinds of breast cancer; they differ in the part of the breast tissue where they originate and in how fast they grow. Most commonly, breast cancer cells kill when they invade other body systems, for example, bones and lungs. Theories about how breast cancer develops are changing. The old theory that cancer starts in the breast, grows and spreads to each of the lymph nodes one by one and then goes to other organs, has not saved lives. The thinking now is that cancer has been in our bodies long before it becomes detectable.

What are the current recommended treatments for breast cancer?

The standard current recommended treatments for breast cancer are a combination of surgery, chemotherapy, and radiation. Surgical treatment can range from radical mastectomy (removal of a breast and adjacent lymph nodes plus chest wall muscles) to lumpectomy (removal of the tumor itself and a small portion of adjacent tissues). Chemotherapy is the administration of combinations of different chemicals either by pills or injections over the course of several months. Radiation is the repeated administration of highly-focused x-rays over a period of time.

These are the treatments authoritatively and strongly advocated by the medical establishment. While there is little compelling evidence of a significant relationship between treatment and survival, they do have immediate effects which are extremely difficult to live with: nausea, exhaustion, lack of ability to concentrate and hair loss. Of the over 200,000 cancer patients receiving chemotherapy annually for all types of cancer, less than 5% can hope for a cure. "Also of concern is the death rate from breast cancer. It hasn't changed in the last 50 years, no matter what advances or changes were made in the treatment." *(A Report on the Women and Cancer Conference, sponsored by the Center for Medical Consumers, and the National Women's Health Network, New York, October 1985.)* Often, 5 years of survival after diagnosis is considered to be a cure. Many women die of breast cancer, 6, 12 or more years after initial diagnosis.

In 1972, the National Cancer Act was passed to provide funding for an all-out war on cancer. After nearly $11 billion has been spent, very little progress has been made except in the treatment of Hodgkins Disease and some leukemias, which are rare cancers. For the major cancer killers of women, advances have been minimal. Surgery is now (in many hospitals) less extensive than it was; lumpectomies are more likely to be done than mastectomies. Chemotherapy is becoming a more popular treatment. For more information on current standard breast cancer treatments, one reasonable source is ***Ourselves, Growing Older***. *(See Resources)*

There are studies which began in 1977 involving tens of thousands of women that seem to show a correlation between reduction in deaths from breast cancer and mammogram screenings in women over age 50. *(See section on mammograms)* The women in these studies are reported to have received standard breast cancer treatments. It is not clear what the results of these studies means. It may be that breast cancer grows at a slower rate in women over 50 or that there may have been treatment of precancerous cells which would never have developed into cancer.

Every person has her own definition of quality of life. Women are encouraged to think about what they are willing to endure as treatment, for how long, and at what expense. It is important to talk to other women who have had breast cancer and breast cancer treatments.

There is very little information available on prevention of breast cancer. There seems to be a correlation between eating fat and the incidence of breast cancer. Reducing the amount of fat that you eat CANNOT HARM YOU! We urge all readers who are concerned about breast cancer to reduce their fat intake considerably.

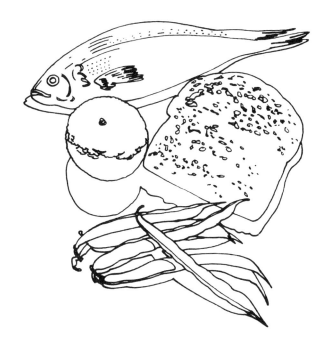

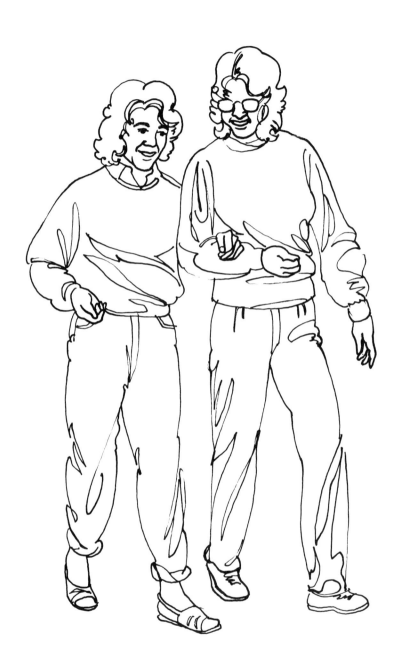

Chapter 8

COMMENTS ON POPULAR SCREENING PROCEDURES: PAP SMEAR, BREAST SELF-EXAM, MAMMOGRAM

Women are big consumers of medical services and, as in other areas, we are always being urged to consume more. Lately women are being pressured to take part in some expensive screening procedures. A screening procedure is one that is done routinely on large numbers of well women, generally with the purpose of detecting disease earlier than it would be detected otherwise. This chapter describes two medical screening procedures, and one that women perform themselves.

Pap Smear

Cervical cancer is a common cancer in women. It may occur at any age, but it occurs most often after age 50.

If a woman has had normal Pap smear results for 3 years in a row, then it is currently thought to be sufficient to have a Pap smear once every 3 years, since cancer of the cervix does not progress rapidly.

During a Pap test, tissue is gently scraped from the cervix and tested for cancer in a laboratory. A woman should not douche before any type of vaginal examination, so as not to change the appearance of the vagina. Pap smears should not be done when a woman has a vaginal infection or during a woman's period, because the results are affected by these two conditions.

It is common practice for clinics and private doctors to notify a patient only if the results of the Pap smear are *not* normal. It is sometimes hard to understand what medical personnel mean when they say something is not "normal." The results of a Pap smear are classified on the basis of the amount of cervical tissue affected, the kinds of cells that are present, and how much they differ from the surrounding cells. The term "dysplasia" is used to mean abnormal cell growth and Cervical Intraepithelial Neoplasia (CIN) describes abnormal cells on or near the cervix.

Pap Smear Classification System

Benign	Absolutely normal or "negative"
Atypical	Not quite normal, either because of infection of another irritation—recommendation: repeat Pap in 3 to 6 months.
CIN I	Intermediate: cells are abnormal, but not
CIN II	necessarily malignant. Recommendation:
CIN III	repeat Pap in 3 to 4 months; if the same class persists, a biopsy should be done. Some doctors will do a biopsy immediately, others take a wait-and-see attitude.
CIN IV	The cells look suspicious for localized cancer. Recommendation: biopsy should be done.

Invasive Cancer

Don't panic if your Pap smear is not normal. Remember, cervical cancer grows very slowly and you have plenty of time to consider all the possibilities.

There is no screening test for uterine cancer. Abnormal bleeding can be a symptom, but is not always one. To be on the safe side, if abnormal bleeding occurs, see your physician for a check-up.

Breast Self-Exam

Breast self-examination has been extensively publicized by those who believe that treatment of tumors detected in this way will result in longer survival. Breast self-exam itself is not harmful. It is the woman herself who is the most likely to find an abnormal condition through regular breast self-exam. A complete description of how to do breast self-examination can be found at the local American Cancer Society, public health department, clinic or in doctors' offices.

Mammograms

There has been a lot of publicity recently about mammograms, which are used as a diagnostic and screening test for breast cancer. Mammograms are x-rays of the breast, and are used to detect cancer. Mammograms are not a treatment or cure for the disease. The American Cancer Society, through the media, doctors, and radiologists, has been urging women to get a so-called base-line mammogram at age 35, and a mammogram every 2 years starting at age 40. The base-line mammogram is for comparison with later mammograms to reveal possible changes in the breast.

However, breasts change throughout a woman's life. When women are in their teens through their thirties, their breasts are dense, making it difficult to see through them with x-rays such as mammograms. As women go through their 40's and 50's, their breast composition changes. After menopause, women's breasts are mostly fatty tissue.

X-rays can see through fat, so mammograms appear to give more accurate information after a woman's menopause. It is difficult to accurately compare mammograms of dense breast tissue at age 35 with mammograms of fatty tissue at age 50. Two studies of large populations of women—comparing those who had mammograms to those who had not—seem to point to a clear reduction in deaths from breast cancer, but only for women over 50 years old. The National Institutes of Health have recommended regular mammograms for women over 50.

Women may ask themselves, can mammograms be harmful?
1. Mammograms usually cost more than $50.
2. Mammograms are x-rays. If a woman starts getting regular mammograms at age 40, by the time she is 70, she will have received 30 years of radiation to a very sensitive area of her body. Radiation can cause cancer. Although the amount of radiation from a mammogram is smaller than it used to be, it is still considered a "high dose" exam.

3. Not all x-ray equipment is in good condition, so the amount of radiation given out may be different from what it is supposed to be. Equipment should be inspected regularly and the person doing the mammogram should be experienced in the proper procedure.
4. There is also the risk of "over-reading" the x-rays. Sometimes tests find areas which are labeled "precancerous" or "preinvasive" because they do not look quite normal, but no one knows if they will grow and become cancerous. For this reason, women have had mastectomies—had their breasts removed—when they did not actually have cancer.

The decision about whether or not to have a mammogram is hard to make because breast cancer is such a frightening disease. The information available is often contradictory and confusing. It is important to trust yourself and to take your time when you make important health care decisions. A woman in tune with her body is the best judge of any changes in her body!

Dose Chart
Average Somatic Doses in Millirads (mrads)
(posing a risk of cancer to the whole body)
from common x-ray examinations.

High-dose Examinations
(more than 125 mrads per average examination):
Mammography (breast exam) .... (250-300)
Upper GI Series (barium swallow) .... (150-400)
Lower GI Series (barium enema, colon exam) .... (90-250)
Lumbosacral spine (lower spine) .... (70-250)
Lumbar spine (lower spine) .... (50-180)

Medium-dose Examinations
(25-125 mrads per average examination):
Intravenous pyelogram, IVP (exam of
kidney & ureter) .... (50-150)
Cervical spine (upper spine) .... (40-80)
Cholecystography (gallbladder exam) .... (25-60)
KUB (kidney, ureter, or bladder exam) .... (10-60)
Skull .... (20-50)
Lumbopelvic (exam of pelvis & lower spine) .... (5-35)

Low-dose Examinations
(less than 25 mrads per average exam):
Chest .... (5-35)
Hip or upper femur (hip or upper thigh exam) .... (2-25)
Shoulder .... (2-25)
Dental (whole mouth or bitewing exam) .... (<5-30)
Extremities (feet, hands, forearms, etc.) .... (<5)

Dose Chart reprinted with permission of The Public Citizen Health Research Group from their *Health Letter*, Volume 3, Number 2, February 1987.

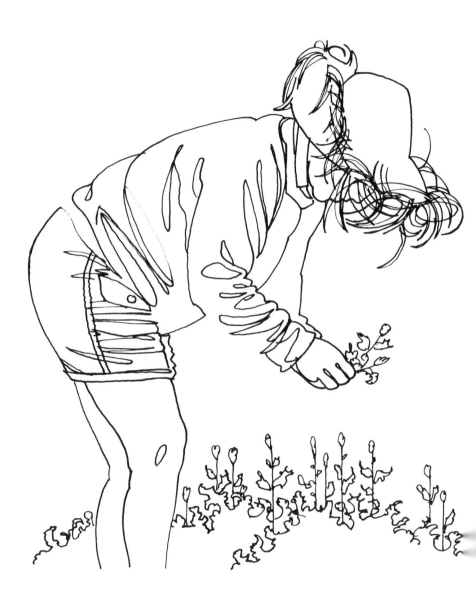

Chapter 9
NATURAL REMEDIES—SELF-HELP

Personal Experience

I had just begun breakthrough bleeding and was told by a gynecologist that I was probably beginning menopause. For that past year my emotions had been out of control and just recently I would cry if someone said "good morning" to me. I searched around and finally at a local herb store got a tincture that addressed the physical and emotional issues and was composed of Dong Quai, hawthorn flowers, black cohosh, and many other vital herbs. It has truly saved my life and helped put me back into balance. I highly recommend it.

When a woman with menopausal complaints goes to see her doctor, chances are that she will be encouraged to use HRT (Hormone Replacement Therapy) and perhaps tranquilizers. Nowadays, however, the safety of this kind of treatment is in question and many women are looking for other ways to get relief. Some of these ways are: a varied diet of fresh foods, herbal remedies, vitamin therapy, and exercise. A woman can try any or all of these on her own, or she can consult a specialist who will set up a program just for her. Specialists who do this kind of work are *curanderas* (herbal healers), herbalists, nutritionists, acupuncturists, chiropractors, naturopaths, and homeopaths.

Herbs

Women all over the world have used herbs (medicinal plants) for menopause signs. We have found the following listed for that purpose: black cohosh, damiana, *dong quai*, cramp bark, *fo-ti-tieng, ginseng*, golden seal, licorice root, red raspberry leaves, sarsaparilla, and *yerba buena* (spearmint). In New Mexico, herbs are often taken in threes, in the belief that a "trinity" has special powers. *Curanderas* prescribe this trinity for hot flashes: *yerba de zorrillo* (worm seed), *escoba de la víbora* (yellow weed or snakeweed), and *yerba del manso* (lizard's tail). Herbalists elsewhere also work with combinations or blends, and so do companies that distribute natural remedies.

Special mention should be made of *ginseng*, a powerful herb that has been used in China for 4,000 years and also is known to Native Americans. It is considered to be a kind of "regulator" which helps the body adjust to unusual conditions, such as heat. It can help with hot flashes, especially when taken with Vitamin E. However, since *ginseng* is very expensive and is sold in a confusing number of products, always buy from a trustworthy store where you can ask for advice on dosages and read the labels carefully. *Dong quai* and *fo-ti-tieng* are other oriental herbs used for women's reproductive health, including the treatment of hot flashes.

Some people recognize and gather wild herbs, while others grow their own. Both methods are good for freshness and economy. Another alternative is to buy them in health food or herb stores. It is important to know the source of the herbs since about 80% of dried herbs sold in the United States come from other countries where pesticides which have been banned in the United States are used. The herbs could have been irradiated or fumigated and there is no way to find out. The ideal situation is to go to a local herbalist who gathers and dries her own herbs.

Herbs are sold both in dried form for making teas and in powdered form (capsules). Most herbs last longer and are fresher if they are not powdered and put into capsules. There are a few exceptions like golden seal, ginger, and slippery elm. Dry herbs should be a color similar to their fresh color, and their scent should be strong. Avoid brown, dull colors and musty and chemical odors when buying herbs.

Up to 6 weeks should be allowed to feel the herbs' effects; do not expect immediate relief. All herbs should be used with caution and started in moderate amounts. Some herbs can be toxic in large amounts. If you are not familiar with an herb, read the labels carefully and ask your supplier for information.

Vitamins and Minerals

The following recommendations on vitamin therapy for menopause signs have been adapted from the book *Women and the Crisis in Sex Hormones* by Barbara Seaman and Gideon Seaman, M.D., and from articles in *Prevention* magazine. One hears of very high dosages of vitamins given to menopausal women by specialists, but remember, these patients are supposed to be closely supervised. For the woman taking vitamins on her own, it is wise to be conservative.

For Hot Flashes: Vitamin E—100-600 units per day—taken after a meal containing some fat. Start with 100 units and gradually increase to 600. Women with diabetes, high blood pressure, or a rheumatic heart condition should not take over 100 units. *People taking digitalis should not take any Vitamin E at all without a doctor's supervision.*

Vitamin E and *ginseng* taken together may give better results than Vitamin E taken alone. Take *ginseng* before meals and Vitamin E after. Do not expect immediate relief; allow up to 6 weeks.

Natural sources of Vitamin E are whole grain breads and cereals, wheat germ (the part of the wheat discarded in milling white flour), nuts, and safflower and wheat germ oils.

For Depression: Feelings of depression and fatigue are often related to specific life events, not to menopause itself. A combination of B vitamins and Vitamin C can be helpful in relieving stress. Health food stores and drug stores carry a variety of "stress formulas" to choose from. They should be taken after breakfast or lunch and not too close to bedtime—they keep some people awake.

Natural sources of the B vitamins are: brewers' yeast, wheat germ, whole grain breads and cereals, and liver. Natural sources of Vitamin C are: citrus fruits, fresh green chile, bell peppers, rose hips, broccoli, and strawberries.

For General Aches and Pains: Calcium can alleviate general aches and pains. Calcium may also help slow down the loss of bone density that comes with aging. The U.S.D.A. recommended daily amount (RDA) of calcium is 800 mg. Researchers now say 1,000 to 1,500 mg per day is better, especially for women past 40. Magnesium and Vitamin D are necessary to help our bodies absorb calcium.

A two-to-one combination of calcium and magnesium is often recommended—1,000 mg of calcium per day and 500 mg of magnesium per day. *(See Chapter 7 on Osteoporosis)* Natural sources of

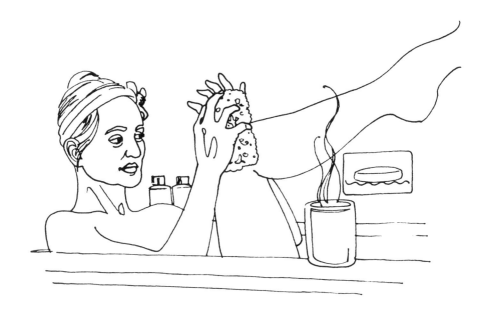

calcium are: milk and milk products (yogurt, cheese, and buttermilk), beets, endive, kale, mustard greens, canned sardines and salmon. Magnesium is found in green leafy vegetables, whole grains, nuts, seeds, and fruits.

Alfalfa leaf tablets are also recommended for joint stiffness and general aches and pains.

For Insomnia: Tryptophan, one of the essential amino acids, is available in tablets. It helps some people with insomnia, and also in some cases with depression. Tryptophan should be taken on an empty stomach and used only as needed, not routinely. Natural sources of tryptophan are milk, meat, and tuna fish.

HOME REMEDIES FOR MENOPAUSE SIGNS
For Hot Flashes

We can learn to live with our hot flashes. First of all, there is no reason to panic—they are natural. Sit down. Take a few deep breaths. Loosen your clothing, or take off a couple of layers. Go outside or stand by an open window. Fan yourself with whatever is at hand. Get something cool to drink. If you have a bedmate —and an electric blanket—get separate controls. Consider telling household members or co-workers what is happening. This is a good time to use your sense of humor. Keep track of hot flashes—notice when they happen and what triggers them. For some women coffee, black tea, sugar, liquor, and spicy foods can trigger hot flashes or make them more intense. Try to minimize or avoid foods and situations that make your flashes more intense. Visualization techniques and biofeedback can also be helpful. Keep track of your hot flashes by writing down when they occur. This may help you see if any specific event triggers them. Other remedies for hot flashes are:

1. Tea from three New Mexico herbs: *yerba de zorrillo* (worm seed), *escoba de la vibora* (yellow weed or snake weed), *yerba del manso* (lizard's tail). Bring half a gallon of water to a boil. Add two tablespoons of dried leaves of each herb (or quarter of a cup of each of the fresh plants, leaves, stems, and roots). Boil 2 to 3 minutes. Set aside covered for 10 minutes. Strain. Drink a cup three times a day.

2. Tea brewed in the same way from two tablespoons of alfalfa seeds to a pint of water. Drink three times a day with lemon. For economy, the same seeds may be used for a second brewing.
3. Dissolve a cup of table salt in a tub of warm water. Lie in it until the water cools. Rinse with cold water and go to bed right away.
   (These three recipes are from Gregorita Rodriguez, Curandera, Santa Fe.)
4. *Dong quai*, also called female *ginseng*, is an oriental herb. A half-inch of *dong quai* root can be kept by your bed and chewed on if you are awakened by hot flashes or night sweats.
5. Tea brewed from wild or sweet marjoram, an ounce in a pint of hot (not boiling) water. Cover. When cool, strain and add a large glass of port wine. Take one teaspoon before meals three times a day.
6. Tea brewed from two parts each of motherwort and red sage, and one part each of tansy, pennyroyal, and skullcap. Take a half-teaspoon in a little lukewarm water before meals three times daily.
7. Tea brewed from black cohosh, sweet flag, licorice root, star root (*aletris arinosa*), black haw, cramp bark (*viburnam opulus*), squaw weed (*false valerian*), and motherwort. Take one cup during the day with a meal.

For Nervousness and/or Sleeplessness

1. Tea brewed from a mixture of catnip, valerian, camomile, skullcap, lady slipper, peppermint.
2. Any one of the following brewed separately as a tea: camomile, skullcap, passion flower (*passiflora incarnata*), tilia flowers.
3. Valerian root in capsules.
4. "Sleepy Time Tea," a blend found in health food stores.
5. Calcium tablets taken at bedtime with hot milk.
6. Tryptophan, one of the essential amino acids. Tablets are for sale in health food stores. (They are expensive.)
7. Sleeping on a pillow stuffed with dried hops.
8. "Calms," an herbal tablet blend (passion flower, hops, camomile).

For Fatigue

Common causes of fatigue, especially among women, are over-work, high stress, undereating, not enough complex carbohydrates, and lack of exercise and fresh air. Most of us do not get sufficient amounts of trace minerals from our daily diets. *Zinc* is an important mineral necessary for hormone metabolism. We should get 25 to 30 mg per day. Natural sources of *zinc* are: meats, whole grains, oysters, herring, clams, peas, and carrots.

Gotu kola is a high mineral herb. Drink one cup of tea in the morning for energy before breakfast. This is not recommended for hyper-thyroid people.

Kelp is a seaweed, a natural source of important minerals such as iodine and potassium, which we often don't get enough of. *Kelp* comes in tablets. One per day, or 150 mg., is recommended for menopausal signs.

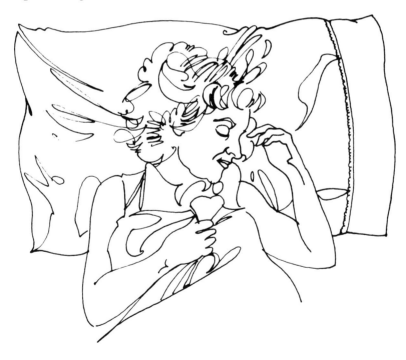

The recipe for home-brew estrogen is free-form and consists of the following steps:

HOME BREW ESTROGEN RECIPE
by Susanne Morgan
(from her book *Coping With a Hysterectomy*,
Dial Press, New York 1982, pp. 177-178. Reprinted with permission.)

EXERCISE
Take, one at a time, two steps toward a better exercise program for you. That might include doing some exercises every day, or it might include adding stretching exercises to walking you already do, or it might include regular running in addition to the stretching or walking you already do. To help produce the home-brew estrogen, you need to improve your exercise program.

NUTRITION
Take two steps toward better nutrition. A good first step for many of us is to eliminate sugar and foods containing sugar. A second step might be to make sure you have fresh fruits and vegetables one more time per day than previously, or to make sure you consume some dairy products each day.

BEVERAGES
Take one step toward reducing your consumption of alcoholic beverages and beverages containing caffeine.

SEXUAL ACTIVITY
Pursue regular sexual activity leading to orgasm and be more active than you have been. This could mean engaging in more sexual activity by yourself, or it could mean a conscious effort to pursue sexual activity with someone else more frequently.

This is the prescription. True, it is easier to take a pill. But the pill will not do nearly as much for us as this prescription will. The pill also may cause problems that we know about now or that may surprise us later.

KEGAL EXERCISES

These exercises are recommended to help reduce dryness of the vagina and to increase enjoyment of intercourse at any age. All the exercises may be continued indefinitely.

How To Do Them

First identify the *pubococcygeus* (PC) muscle you are trying to strengthen:

Sit on the toilet. Spread your legs as far apart as possible, then start and stop the flow of urine. The PC muscle is the only one that can accomplish this while in this position.

Once a woman learns where the muscle is, the Kegel exercises can be done during daily activities such as driving an automobile, sitting, doing dishes, watching television, or lying in bed.

Exercise 1

Contract the PC muscle, hold for 3 seconds, relax and repeat the process. These may be done as often during the day as desired, but approximately 90 contractions (six 1-minute periods each day) are recommended. With too strenuous exercise, the PC muscle can become sore. If this happens, either stop doing the exercises for 1 or 2 days until the temporary soreness disappears then resume, or reduce the number done per day and then gradually increase.

Exercise 2

Contract and release the PC muscle very rapidly, 25 to 50 times a day (10 contractions at a time). Although the contractions during orgasm are much more rapid, this exercise approximates what the PC muscle does during orgasm.

Exercise 3

This exercise involves bearing down as if trying to expel a baby during labor. With this exercise, it has been demonstrated that the blood supply to the genitals increases, with a consequent increase of lubrication in the vagina. For 3 seconds (holding to a count of three), bear down, relax, and repeat. Do 25 to 50 times daily.

Exercise 4

Raise the entire pelvic area as though sucking water into the vagina. Insert a finger and feel the vagina drawing it in. Do 25 to 50 times daily.

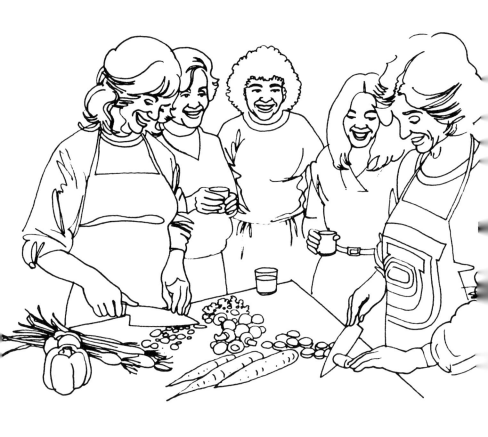

Chapter 10
NUTRITION

With age, recovery from physical exertion and stress usually takes longer. At the same time, it may be harder to get a good night's sleep. In other words, there seems to be less margin for overdoing things, and the return to normal is slower. For this reason, taking good care of the body becomes more important than ever. Many people also find that metabolism and activity levels change. This means that women need to stay active in order to maintain their weight, and it becomes very important to make quality food choices. Eating a variety of foods, especially fresh vegetables and fruit, whole grains, and small amounts of fat, will result in a higher energy level and a greater sense of well-being.

If a woman pays attention to how foods make her feel, she can start eliminating or cutting back on foods which do not agree with her. For example, some bodies may be less tolerant of some things, like caffeine, fatty cuts of meat, or spicy foods. Other things to be careful of are "hidden" ingredients such as pesticides, chemicals, sugar, salt, and fat. These ingredients are added to processed foods to make them appear fresh for a longer time. In general, processed foods are less nutritious than fresh foods, and have extra calories, fats, and health risks.

Sometimes it is difficult to make good choices about what to eat. There is little public or media pressure about eating healthy foods, and people make more money by processing foods than they do by leaving them in their natural state.

Read the labels on food containers to find out what you are really eating. The more ingredients you don't recognize, the more processed the food has been. For example, canned vegetables have fewer nutrients than frozen vegetables, which in turn have fewer nutrients than fresh ones.

This chapter presents basic information on nutrition and some suggestions for those who are interested in changing eating habits.

Suggestions for Change

1. Write a list of everything you have eaten in the last 24 hours, or longer. Then set up a page with the five food categories described below. Write down what you ate under the appropriate category. Don't forget to write down all ingredients; for example a salad made up of lettuce, tomatos, avocado, blue cheese, oil, and vinegar would be listed under vegetables and fats. When you look at the chart, you may see some unexpected patterns. For example, are there foods that you like, but didn't eat? Did you list many foods under fats and "others"?

2. Food preparation is an area where healthy choices can be made. If others in the household are big milk drinkers, you can make a gradual change to low-fat and then to skim milk. You can try more roasted or baked foods instead of fried ones.

3. In our workshops, when we ask people to name the food they like to eat best, they most frequently name healthy foods. Think of adding to meals foods that you like, which are nutritionally good. For example, a mother who buys oranges and milk for her children may decide that she deserves them too.

4. Healthier foods can be substituted for some not-so-healthy foods. Some people like to drink diluted hot apple juice instead of coffee during the winter months, and fruit juices diluted with carbonated water instead of soft drinks when it's hot . If you don't spend money buying high sugar, salt, or fat foods, there may be extra money to buy your favorite fruits.

5. Try eating *less* of some foods such as fat, salt, sugar, caffeine, and alcohol, instead of saying you can *never* eat them. When you eat less of foods high in such ingredients, you may have less interest in them. Popcorn might easily be enjoyed without salt or butter, but soup may still be better with some salt. A bite of dessert can be enjoyed without eating a whole serving.

6. Read food labels carefully, they have all sorts of useful information on them. For example, the low-fat yogurt with fruit label can tell us that the calories taken out of the yogurt in the fat were returned with the sugar in the fruit.

Food Categories

It is helpful to be aware of major food categories. Everyone needs a variety of whole grains, vegetables, fruits, and animal protein foods. Most people eat more fats and "other" foods than they need.

1. A variety of grains or complex carbohydrates in their natural unrefined form contain protein, vitamins and minerals. Examples of these foods are: brown rice, dried beans, corn, whole grain noodles, and potatoes. Most of the world gets the bulk of its nourishment from such complex carbohydrates. They are relatively inexpensive.

2. Vegetables and fruits also are carbohydrates which contain vitamins and minerals. They are needed to help our bodies absorb the foods we eat. Long periods of cooking reduce the nutrients in vegetables.

3. Animal protein foods are also useful to build body tissues. Animal foods which are especially high in complete protein are: chicken, turkey, fish, eggs, meat, cheese, and milk. Most people in the United States eat too much of these high protein foods, which also contain a lot of fat. Small amounts of these animal protein foods, combined with complex carbohydrates, give us complete proteins with less fat. Examples are: beans and rice, noodles and spaghetti sauce, and chicken and rice. Animal protein foods are relatively expensive.

4. Fats store up energy. Foods high in fat are: butter, margarine, lard, oils, and bacon. Other fatty foods are: cheese, red meat, whole milk, nuts, and avocados. Fat has more than twice as many calories per unit of weight as carbohydrates do. A body does need fat, but almost everyone takes in much more than she actually needs.

5. "Other" foods are those which have little or no nutritive value. Many processed foods, salty fried snacks and sweets belong in this category. Other items in this category are: coffee, black tea, soft drinks, alcohol, sugar, chewing gum, potato chips, ice cream, ketchup and mustard.

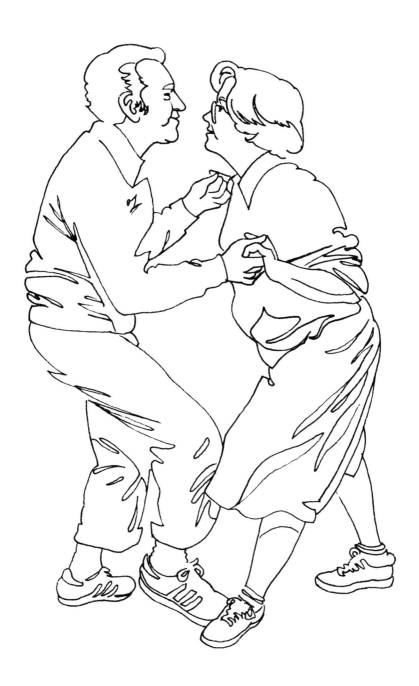

Chapter 11
EXERCISE

Personal Experience

I didn't want to take estrogen, and it didn't agree with me. The only other thing the doctor recommended was exercise. My sister-in-law said, why don't you walk with us? I went every day early in the morning. Within a week's time I was able to sleep through the night, which I hadn't been able to do in a long time because of the hot flashes and everything.

Not a day passes without an article in the newspapers telling how exercise is the cure for another disease—diabetes, hypertension, heart trouble, back problems—and the list goes on. There is controversy about many of these findings, but one thing is obvious: people do feel better when they exercise. It helps them sleep, eat, think, and lose weight. Exercise is something our ancestors took for granted, but in the modern world, office jobs, washing machines, supermarkets, and automobiles have taken away exercise as a part of daily living.

When a person exercises, most of the body muscles get a workout, but one muscle, the heart, works harder than any of the others. Its job of sending fresh blood and oxygen to all parts of the body is increased during exercise. And, like all muscles, the more it is used, the bigger and stronger it gets. Regular exercise will make the heart work more efficiently. A person who exercises regularly has a slower heart beat at rest than a person who does not exercise regularly.

Any exercise that lasts longer than 20 minutes without making you "huff and puff" is good. (If you can carry on a conversation as you exercise, you are doing it at the appropriate level. If you cannot talk, slow down; if you can sing, you are going too slow). Long-distance running, jogging, swimming, bicycling, fast walking, cross-country skiing and jumping rope are all good exercises. However, start to train your body slowly, so that it gets used to this new routine. Do not decide to go out and run for 20 minutes one day when you have never done it before.

Before beginning any exercise program, think for a moment. Do you have any health problems? If so, then you should check with your doctor before starting.

Start your program slowly, building up the strength of your heart and breathing capacity of your lungs. Work up to more strenuous effort as your heart and muscles become used to this new activity.

In any exercise program it is very important to begin by warming up sufficiently so that muscles or joints will not be hurt. Flexibility exercises will help you avoid injury in strenuous exercises, and generally prepare your body for action. It takes people different amounts of time to get their bodies ready for stenuous exercises.

After doing various stretching exercises for 5 to 10 minutes, begin your strenuous exercise, but start slowly. Do the exercise for a short period of time, then, as the weeks progress, begin to build up the exercise time to make your body work harder. For instance, a walking program could begin with walking 1 mile, five times a week, for 20 minutes. You may need to start your program more slowly by walking four times a day for 5 minutes at a time or twice a day for 10 minutes. After you can comfortably walk for 20 minutes at a time, your next goal might be to increase the amount of time you walk. Finally, you could practice walking faster for the same period of time. You might go from walking a mile in 20 minutes to walking a mile-and-a-half in 30 minutes. Then, try to cover a mile-and-three-quarters in 30 minutes over a course of several weeks. Continue this schedule regularly at the time and pace that is right for you.

The same could be done with a bicycle. For example, you could start with 3 flat miles, five times a week, for 20 minutes each time. Increase to 5 miles in 25 minutes the next week. Then try 6 miles in 35 minutes the third week, and so on.

To begin a running program, you could start the first week with walking and running a mile. Try to do it in 18 minutes. The second week try a mile in 16 minutes. The third week try for 15 minutes. This should be done four times a week, then begin to add an extra half-mile. For the next few weeks strive to bring your time down. This type of schedule can also be followed for swimming, racquetball, handball, squash, jumping rope, or running in place.

After exercising, you need a cooling off period to get your body back to its normal heart rate. Do not just stop the exercise and sit down. Allow your body to adjust or you could have a dizzy spell, or even faint. Five minutes of walking slowly or very slow jogging will bring your body back to normal.

These invigorating exercises are called aerobic (with oxygen) exercises because they increase heart and lung activity for a long time and will help make conditioning changes in the body.

In any program, the first 6 weeks are the hardest. Your frame of mind is an important part of conditioning. Promise yourself to stick with the program for 8 weeks and after that time you will begin to enjoy it and notice a pleasant change. You will begin to look forward to your exercise and feel bad if you do not do it.

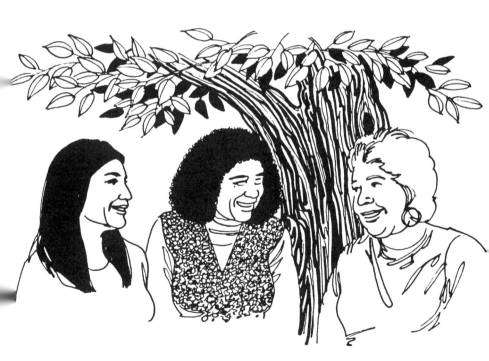

A Final Note

We hope this book will help you to become more questioning users of health information, services and products, more critical listeners to health practicioners, the media and friends, and stronger as women in today's sexist and ageist society. One way we have found to help ourselves do these things is to be part of a group, to talk with each other, sometimes informally, sometimes in organized groups. Nothing makes you feel less crazy than being in a group and learning that others experience the same things.

We would appreciate hearing your reactions to our book and to your menopause. We are glad to have been part of the movement to bring menopause out of the closet. We hope you will join us.

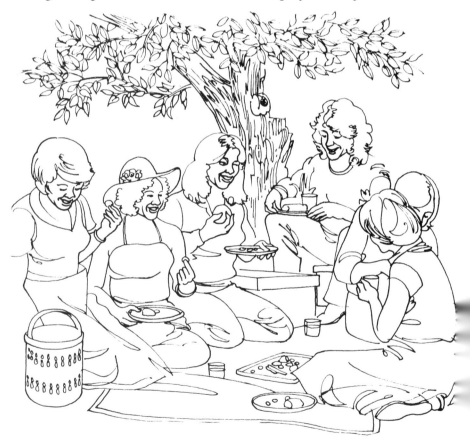

The lists below are highly selective. *References* are the materials that were used to help write the text. *Resources* are additional materials on related topics. Although there are other widely available books on the subjects covered in this manual, they are not listed here because the authors do not feel they add pertinent information to the topics discussed in this manual.

References

Books

Boston Women's Health Book Collective, *The New Our Bodies, Ourselves*, Simon & Schuster, Inc.: New York, 1984. Paperback. An excellent general book for women about their bodies.

Brody, Jane, *Jane Brody's Nutrition Book.* W.W. Norton & Company: New York, 1981. Clear, complete, basic nutrition book, includes recipes.

Dorland's Illustrated Medical Dictionary. 26th Edition, W.B. Saunders Company: Philadelphia, 1981. A useful reference for medical terminology.

Hatcher, Robert A., M.D. et al., *Contraceptive Technology 1988-1989.* Irvington Publishers, Inc.: New York, 1988. Comprehensive reference book on contraception, updated annually.

Lesbian Health Matters, A Santa Cruz Women's Health Collective Publication, Santa Cruz, CA., 1979. One of the few women's health books written particularly for Lesbians.

McCauley, Carole Spearin, *Pregnancy After 35.* Pocket Books: New York, 1976. Practical information for future middle-aged mothers.

Doress, Paula Brown, and Diana Laskin Siegal, et al., *Ourselves, Growing Older.* Simon & Schuster, Inc.: New York, 1987. Uses some material on menopause written by the Santa Fe Health Education Project; covers a wide range of topics.

Montreal Health Press, Editors, *Birth Control Handbook.* 12th ed. rev. Montreal Health Press, C.P. 1000, Station Place du Parc: Montreal, Quebec, Canada H2W 2N1 1985. Comprehensive, easy-to-read guide to contraception, a pamphlet.

Morgan, Susanne, *Coping With a Hysterectomy.* Dial Press: New York, 1982. Contains some useful information and strong personal opinions.

Nissim, Rina, *Natural Healing in Gynecology, A Manual for Women.* English Edition. Pandora Press in association with Methuen Inc.: 29 West 35th Street, New York, 10001, 1986. A guide for natural healing of gynecological problems.

Reitz, Rosetta, *Menopause: A Positive Approach.* Penguin Books: New York, 1979. Women 25 to 95 years of age talk about sex and aging, male menopause, nutrition, estrogen, and more.

Rose, Louisa, Editor, *The Menopause Book.* Hawthorn Books: New York, 1977. Eight women doctors provide answers to medical questions which affect middle-age women. The section on sex at menopause is especially helpful.

Seaman, Barbara and Gideon Seaman, M.D., *Women and the Crisis in Sex Hormones.* Bantam: New York 1978. The most comprehensive information on the side effects of estrogen and birth control methods, and wholesome remedies for menopause complaints. It is a little dated, but the information is still relevant.

Weed, Susan, *Wise Woman Herbal for the Child-Bearing Years.* Ash Tree Publishing: P.O. Box 64, Woodstock, New York, 12498, 1986. Many herbs used in this book are also helpful to the menopausal woman.

Articles
Advances in Nursing Science, July 1985. MacPherson, Kathleen I., "Osteoporosis and Menopause: A Feminist Analysis of the Social Construction of a Syndrome."

A Friend Indeed Publication, Vol. III, No. 7, 1986. "The Great Hormone Debate."

Health Facts, Center for Medical Consumers, New York, NY, Vol. XIII, No. 110, July, 1988. "A Critical Look at the New Chemotherapy Recommendations."

Health Facts, Center for Medical Consumers, New York, NY, Vol VIII No. 55 December 1983. "On Accepting Medical Pronouncements,"

Health Facts, Center for Medical Consumers, New York, NY, Vol. XI, No. 91, December 1986. "Trends in Surgery."

Health Letter, Public Citizen Health Research Group, Washington, D.C., Vol. 3, No. 2, February, 1987, "Dose Charts."

Health Letter, Public Citizen Health Research Group, Washington D.C., Vol. 3, No. 5, May, 1987. "Osteoporosis Part One: Screening Tests."

Health Letter, Public Citizen Health Research Group, Vol. 3, No. 6, June 1987, "Osteoporosis Part Two: Prevention and Treatment."

Journal of American Medical Association, Vol. 259, No. 10, March 11, 1988. Bailar, John, M.D., "Mammogram Before Age 50 Years?"

Network News, The Publication of the National Women's Health Network, July/August, 1988, "Osteoporosis: Sorting Fact from Fallacy."

Newsweek, April 11, 1977."Smoking and the Pill."

Reports

A Report from the Women and Cancer Conference, "Breast Cancer," Oct. 26, 1985. Edited by Maryann Napoli, Center for Medical Consumers, 237 Thompson St., New York, 10025 (212)674-7105.

Consensus Conference, "Osteoporosis," *Journal of the American Medical Association,* Aug. 10, 1984, Vol. 252, No. 6, pp.799-802.

"Statement of Public Citizen Health Research Group before the National Institutes of Health Consensus Development Conference on Osteoporosis," April 2-4, 1984. National Institutes of Health, Bethesda, Maryland, page 2 of the transcript.

Periodicals

Broomstick, Options for Women Over 40, 3543 18th St. #3, San Francisco, CA 94110.

Hot Flash, Newsletter of the National Action Forum for Midlife & Older Women, c/o Jane Porcino, Box 816, Stony Brook, NY 11790-0609.

Nutrition Action, Health Letter of the Center for Science in the Public Interest, 1501 16th St. NW, Washington D.C. 20036-1499.

Resources

Organizations

A Friend Indeed, Inc., Les publications une véritable amie, inc. Box 515, Place du Parc Station, Montréal, Quebac H2W2Pl (514) 843-5730.

Boston Women's Health Book Collective, 47 Nichols St., Watertown, MA 02172, (617)924-0271. Packets of information on many health topics available.

National Women's Health Network. 1325 G Street NW, Washington D.C. 20005.

Santa Fe Health Education Project, P.O.Box 577, Santa Fe, NM 87504-0577, (505)983-3236.

Book

Hemphill, Delores and Yvonne Kimber, *A Positive Look at Menopause*. Teacher Training Manual, Planned Parenthood of Central Missouri, 800 North Providence, Suite 11, Columbia, MO 65201.

ABBREVIATIONS AND TERMS USED IN THIS MANUAL

CIN - Cervical Intraepithelial Neoplasia describes abnormal cells on or near the cervix.

Dalkon Shield - an intrauterine contraceptive device no longer on the market.

DES - Diethylstilbestrol is a synthetic estrogen.

D&C - Dilation and Curettage describes the dilation of the cervix and the scraping out of the lining of the uterus.

ERT - Estrogen Replacement Therapy is the taking of additional estrogen as prescribed by doctors.

Estrogen - a generic term for a group of female sex hormones. In women estrogen is formed in the ovaries, adrenal cortex, and the fat cells.

FSH - Follicle Stimulating Hormone is one of the female sex hormones regulated by the pituitary gland and affecting the menstrual cycle.

HRT - Hormone Replacement Therapy is the taking of additional estrogen and progesterone as prescribed by doctors.

Induced Menopause - menopause brought on by outside influences such as surgery, chemotherapy, and radiation.

LH - Luteinizing Hormone is one of the female sex hormones produced in the ovaries.

Progesterone - a female sex hormone produced in the ovaries, adrenal cortex, and the placenta.

RDA - Recommended Daily Allowance is the abbreviation that is used to indicate how much of a nutrient is recommended.

U.S.D.A. - United States Department of Agriculture, which sets standards for the daily intake of a wide variety of nutrients.

Need More Copies?
Use coupon below or call (505) 982-3236.
Discounts available
for bulk or dealer orders.

- -

Santa Fe Health Education Project
P.O. Box 577
Santa Fe, New Mexico 87504-0577
Phone (505) 982-3236

Please send _____ copies of **Menopause Manual** at $5 per copy plus $1.50 postage/handling.

Enclosed is check or money order for $_____ payable to Santa Fe Health Education Project.

Name_____

Address_____

City_____State_____Zip_____